The Joys of Etiquette

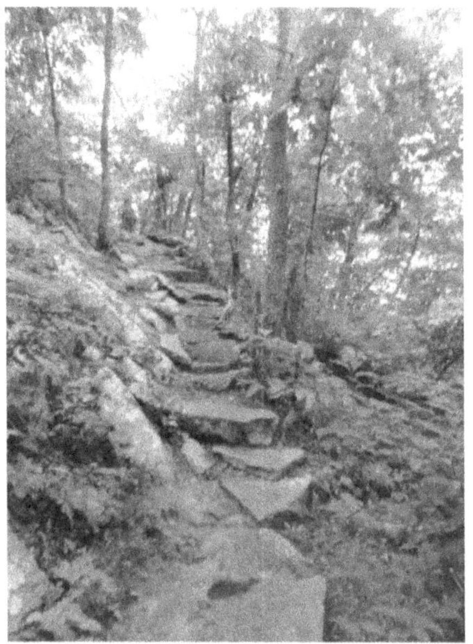

Hiking Edition

by Sandy Balliet

Sandra Balliet

The Joys of Etiquette – Hiking Edition

Copyright © 2022 by Sandra Balliet

All rights reserved. No part of this publication may be reproduced, stored or transmitted in any form or by any means, electronic, mechanical, photocopying, recording, scanning, or otherwise without written permission from the publisher. It is illegal to copy this book, post it to a website, or distribute it by any other means without permission.

This novel is entirely a work of fiction. The names, characters and incidents portrayed in it are the work of the author's imagination. Any resemblance to actual persons, living or dead, events or localities is entirely coincidental.

Sandra Balliet asserts the moral right to be identified as the author of this work.

Sandra Balliet has no responsibility for the persistence or accuracy of URLs for external or third-party Internet Websites referred to in this publication and does not guarantee that any content on such Websites is, or will remain, accurate or appropriate.

Designations used by companies to distinguish their products are often claimed as trademarks. All brand names and product names used in this book and on its cover are trade names, service marks, trademarks and registered trademarks of their respective owners. The publishers and the book are not associated with any product or vendor mentioned in this book. None of the companies referenced within the book have endorsed the book.

First edition

This book was professionally typeset on Reedsy
Find out more at reedsy.com

Contents

1.

2.

3.

4.

5.

6.

1

Introduction

Are you thinking about getting out and enjoying the great outdoors? That is great, but there are a few unwritten rules you need to follow that you are courteous to other hikers and a good steward to nature.

- Rule number 1: Don't get lost. Make sure you have a reliable map and know how to read it.
- Rule number 2: Know what to do if you do get lost

Virtually every group of people will have written and unwritten rules to help manage their activity and make things more enjoyable for those participating. Rules such as no tailgating on the highway, not butting in line no matter where you are, and keeping your mouth closed while chewing while having a meal are good manners.

The hiking community is no different. Following the unwritten rules can help make your hike and the hike for others more enjoyable. Following are several observed hiking etiquette practices:

2

Know your right of way

So, do you think you are ready to go out in the great wilderness and go hiking? Well, do you have boots that fit your feet? Have you broken them in by walking around the house and neighborhood? If not, please go to a hiking store and get fitted properly for shoes made for the trails. Please take my word for it; getting blisters while hiking in the incorrect shoes is no fun. Take a pack with you to put your water, snacks, first aid kit, and any other necessities you think you will need. Do you have trekking poles? No, you might want to invest in a pair; they come in handy when crossing streams or going up and down hills. Do you ever get confused about who has the right-of-way on multi-use trails? Should you move aside for bikes, or are they supposed to watch out for hikers and horses? What is the etiquette when meeting up with a horse on the trail? You would be surprised how many beginner and experienced hikers do not know the right-of-way to follow. Well, you can first check to see if there is a bulletin board at the trailhead with information and maps. The bulletin board is where you should see a right-of-way yield sign. Otherwise, here is a guide for you to follow.

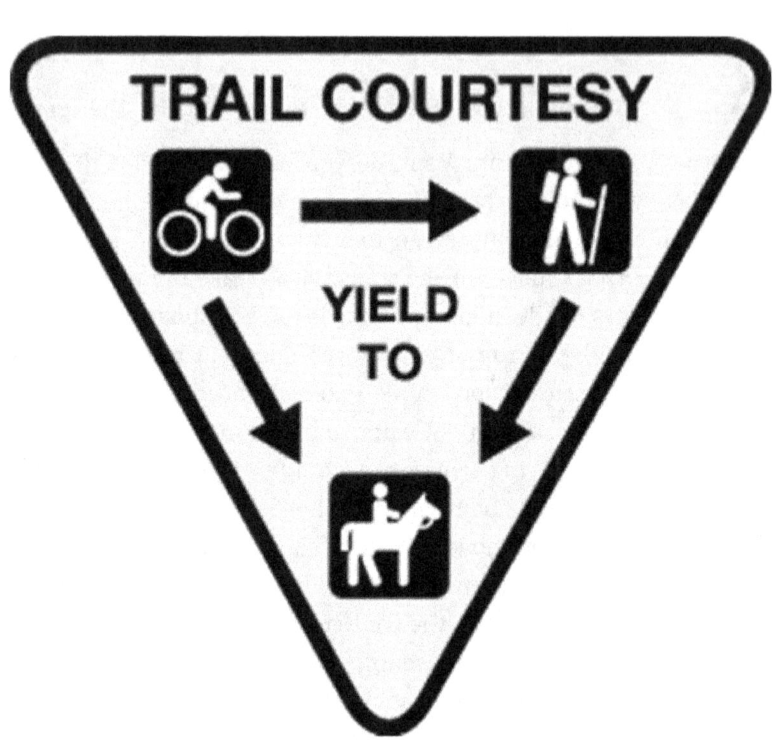

TRAIL COURTESY
YIELD
TO

Hikers vs. Bikers: Since bikes are considered more maneuverable than hikers' legs, bikers, generally, are to yield to hikers on the trail. However, this isn't always the case because bikes often move faster than hikers' legs can carry them. Usually, it is simpler and easier for hikers to yield the right of way—especially if a biker is gasping and wheezing up a challenging hill or coming around a blind curve. But this can give some people the wrong idea about who has the right of way. A biker should not expect a hiker to yield, and bikers need to be extra cautious and anticipate what's up ahead on the trail. Because bikers move faster, hikers should also be aware of their surroundings on shared trails. Conscientious bikers will call out or ring a bell as they ride around blind switchbacks or down steep slopes and should also let you know how many other bikers are following them.

Hikers vs. Horses: As the (usually) slowest-to-maneuver, least-predictable, and largest domestic animals on the trail, horses have the right-of-way from both hikers and bikers. If you're sharing the trail with horseback riders, give them as wide a berth as possible, make sure not to make unexpected movements as they pass, and talk calmly when approaching to avoid frightening the animal. When you're on a narrow trail and horses (or mules) are passing, get off the trail on the downhill side as they pass you. When spooked, Horses are more likely to run uphill than downhill. You want to be out of the way of a spooked horse. Take care when coming up behind a horse. Horses cannot see directly behind themselves, so approaching from behind can be hazardous to both the horse and the hiker or biker. Horses may kick out in what they perceive as self-defense. Communication is critical in these situations: gently announce yourself in advance, let the horse and rider know that you are hiking up from behind, and ask/wait for direction from the rider. It pays to be cautious and safe when on the trail.

Bikers vs. Horses: Remember, if you are on a bike, it is your responsibility to yield to hikers and horses. The thought is that bikers are potentially fast and could come into conflict if passing horses and hikers too quickly. Bikers should slow down when coming upon hikers or horses; when going downhill, preferable stop and let the hikers pass them by. Bikers can stop and go quickly; thus, they give other users the right of way. Horses are big and unpredictable, so horses always have the right way. Horses, riders, and hikers have also been hurt by bikers while also risking severe injury for themselves. Bikers can be charged and held criminally liable for any injuries they cause in these cases. So, know the right-of-way and be cautious of your speed.

Hikers vs. Hikers: It looks as if many hikers—even the most experienced ones—may not know or always remember this, but the accepted agreement is that hikers going uphill have the right of way. The reasoning is that a hiker going up a trail will have a shorter range of vision and not see those ahead of them. Another reason may be in that "hiking rhythm" zone and may not want to stop their pace. Often an uphill hiker will take a break to rest their legs and catch their breath or get a drink to let others pass come downhill. Remember that's the hiker going uphill's decision. If you're coming up to another hiker from behind and wish to pass, announce your presence, a simple "hello" is often the best. Many hikers get into the "zone" while going up long inclines.

Always hike single file, never taking up more than half the trail space; the only time it is acceptable to hike beside someone is when the trail is wide enough to accommodate more people hiking in both directions. Hiking in large groups can get loud and crowded on the trails, which makes it harder for someone to pass them. Limiting groups to 10 or less is recommended; it is better for the trails and easier for others to go around. Please stay on the trail itself when hiking or passing others. Those off-trail boot prints, over time, can badly erode hills and switchbacks and destroy drainage diversions. Should Solo Hikers Move for Big Groups? The answer is yes. Especially if the large group is following proper trail etiquette and hiking in single file to not go off trail and risk trampling plants and wildlife, and yes, wildlife includes insects. As a solo hiker or in a small group, it's easier to step aside and let the group pass.

Trail etiquette is even more important if you are hiking in a group. If you can see that your pace is faster than the hiker(s) ahead of you, you will have to catch up and then pass this hiker. Passing can be a tricky proposition; newer hikers don't think about yielding the right of way to anyone behind them. Other times, hikers can be deep in conversation and not hear someone approaching from behind. It's also possible that the hiker you are approaching could be hard of hearing, or they could be wearing earbuds and not hear you. Another consideration is the sound of nature bird calls, moving water, and the wind.

Just remember, bikers yield to both hikers and horses, and hikers yield to horses. Horses have the right-a-way all the time. When passing, the same rules apply as when driving a car: stay to the right and pass on the left.

When in doubt, treat anyone you meet on the trail the same way you'd treat the trail —with respect. Then get back to enjoying the solitude and quiet of the trail.

3

Leave No Trace

The Leave no trace principle is easy to leave nature, well, natural. We are all guests in nature, and you want to be a good guest. When hiking, you will wish to bring some water and food or snacks with you; however, you need to remember that hiking trails usually do not have a trash can on them, so don't toss your trash – not even biodegradable items such as apple cores. Who wants to wade through trash while hiking? If you packed it to go in with you, pack it back out with you. Below you will find the seven leave no trace principles that everyone who enjoys the outdoors should be following;

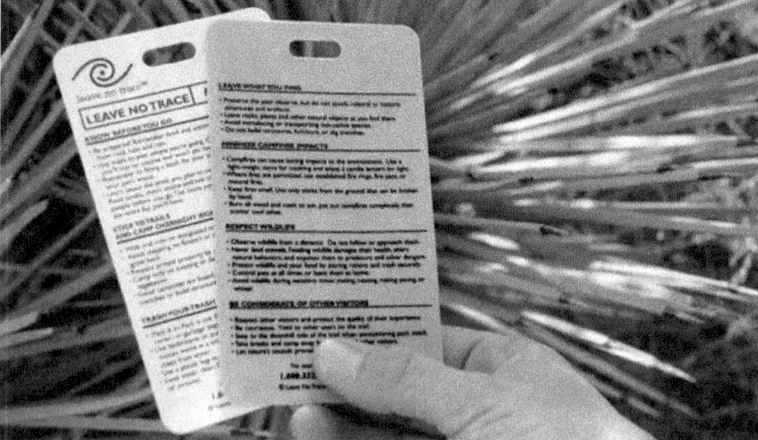

1. Plan and prepare ahead of time. Research Park rules and tail information. Check with the closest forest service for

fire restrictions. Research the trail and keep a map with you. Check the weather before you leave, learn of weather conditions you might run into, and prepare for all conditions. Check your maps to know the terrain you will be hiking. Hike in small groups of 10 or less to minimize the impact on the trail and avoid high use times. Walking in a single file and avoiding shortcuts will limit damage to the trail and surrounding ecosystems.

2. Travel and camp on durable surfaces. Focus on hiking and camping on durable ground. Durable ground includes gravel, sand, rock, dry grass, and snow. These surfaces can best withstand heavy use. Surfaces such as marshes, bogs, and alpine meadows are too fragile to withstand heavy foot traffic. Walk through mud/puddles, and not around, to avoid widening the trail. Spread out so you will avoid making new trails when hiking in a place with no noticeable trail. Camp in designated areas and try to be at least 200ft away from water. If there is no designated area to camp, minimize your impact by camping on gravel, dry grass, or snow. Camping close to water sources can disrupt animals' access or could cause conflict with you.

3. Dispose of waste properly. Pack it in, pack it out! This includes food wrappers and biodegradable waste such as apple cores, eggshells, etc. These can take months before biodegrading, all the while attracting animals. The last thing you need is animals drawn to your camp looking for handouts. Just think, if a skunk is looking for easy food and you scare it, whew no one will want to be near you, yourself included. Also, practice "negative trace" by bringing an extra bag to pick up trash left by others. When possible, make use of pit toilets and outhouses. Move at least 200 feet away from any water source to dispose of human waste; dig your cathole 6–8 inches

deep in the soil. Take out all toilet paper and hygiene products; do not bury them.

4. Leave what you find. You can look, but please leave everything you find in the wilderness where it belongs. Do not move rocks, pick plants, or disturb cultural or historical artifacts. This allows others to enjoy the trails in the same condition you found them. Take pictures to enjoy later and leave the flowers and rocks where you found them. Many insects, bugs, and animals live under rocks, and when you disturb the rock, you destroy their homes. Rocks are also used as trail markers, and moving the rocks from these markers can detrimentally affect a hiker, making them lost or confused.

5. Minimize campfire impacts. Campfires can have negative impacts on the soil. Keep your campfire small—or go without. Check with the fire service before leaving to know the area's danger level. Use previously constructed fire rings or mounds. Only burn small wood found on the ground that is dead to avoid harming trees. Do not cut live trees and leave fallen trees where they are; they significantly benefit the ecosystem. Make sure your campfire is smothered before you leave camp, spread your coals, drown them in water, and cover them with dirt. Even the tiniest spark can start a forest fire. Small camping/backpacking stoves are much more efficient for cooking and leave no impact on the camping site.

6. Respect wildlife. Watch and don't interact with wildlife; keep your distance. You want to stay at least 200 yards away from most wildlife. Please do not feed or bait them with food intended for human consumption, as this disrupts their natural foraging habits and may harm them. Some human foods can be deadly to animals. Never leave food unattended; store all food in a bear canister, a food locker, or properly hang from a tree. Control pets in

natural areas and keep them restrained; don't let them constantly chase or bark at wildlife.

7. People experience the wilderness in various ways, some for fitness, some for spending time in nature, and some for socializing. Be considerate of other visitors. Please show respect for others and don't let your experience negatively affect theirs. Keep voices/noises from getting intrusively loud. Step away from the trail when taking rest breaks for photo shots. Situate rest spots and campsites away from the trail. Try to minimize visual impacts by wearing clothes that are earth tone colors (unless hiking during hunting season): brown, green, tan, or black.

4

What is Trail Etiquette for Dogs?

Going on a hike and taking your dog is an excellent way for both to get some exercise and fresh air. Remember, even your pup isn't exempt from the trail rules! If a trail has a leash rule, consider the following:

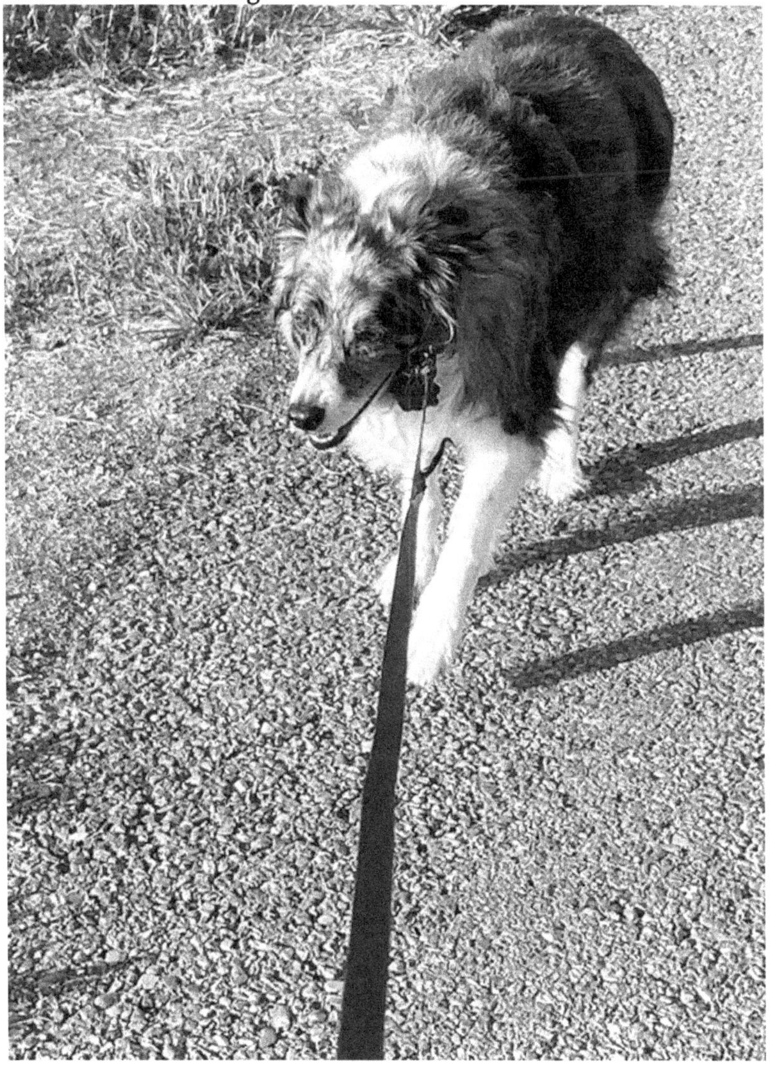

Not everyone likes dogs. I know it's astonishing; dogs are some of the best people I know. Some people are terrified of dogs. Many say that dogs walking off-leash on trails makes it difficult and scary because it throws them off balance. Even if your dog is well-behaved, it may ruin a nervous walker's day. The last thing you want to do is ruin someone's enjoyment of the outdoors with your dog.

Dogs, even the most well-behaved ones, love to chase wildlife and birds. Think of the squirrels that dogs love to try and catch. Many trails go right through extraordinary habitats and nesting areas. These areas could be fragile, or the wildlife will not nest in areas that dogs are known to run in. Think of nesting peregrine falcons with special nesting boxes, and if a dog finds these boxes, the falcons might abandon their nests with eggs or babies in them. They may disturb their habitat even if your dog isn't chasing the animals or birds. It is best to constantly watch your dog, ensuring they are not disturbing any wildlife.

You're probably thinking, I always pick up after my dog. But if your dogs are off leash and running in the tall grass, you have no idea what they're doing. When your dog is off-leash and not in direct eyesight, you may not notice that they're pooping, and you'll miss picking up after them. Refer to our last post; pick up two poos next time.

Not every dog can be off leash, so their owners will walk them on a leash. If your off-leash dog approaches another on-leash dog, there can be conflict. You might think your dog is very friendly to all, but if the dog they are running up to is not, you are causing unnecessary conflict between the owner and their dog. Before allowing your dog to approach another person or dog, ask to see if they are OK with being approached and follow their orders on this. Be respectful to other dog owners and keep your on-leash or right at your side, so they don't have to worry about unleashed dogs approaching.

Children can be toppled easily by unleashed dogs, even the well-behaved ones. Children or dogs can be enthusiastic and not realize they could hurt each other.

Unleashed wandering dogs can trample native plants and rare wildflowers. When leashed, the dogs stay on trial, keeping them on the trail so we can continue to enjoy the beautiful flora and fauna.

If the dogs are on trails that allow off-leash play, always keep your dog in eyesight and under control. With dogs off-leash, you have perfect voice command over your dog, and they come whenever called. When approaching other hikers, keep your dog under control at your side and step to the side of the trail.

Pay attention to your dog

Please do not let your dog wander out of sight; keep them on the trail and clean up after them; chasing and barking at the wildlife should not be allowed or trampling through flora and fauna. Please be considerate and don't leave your poop bags lying around for others to pick up (even if you intend to pick the poop bag up on the way out). The last thing someone who is hiking wants to do is skirt around piles of dog poo or poo bags.

5

Be Friendly to Other Hikers

Make yourself known. Just because you're having a great time bagging peaks and taking names doesn't mean being friendly and chatty with other hikers you meet on the trail isn't essential, especially if you are hiking alone or have a long route. Stopping to say hello and chat with fellow hikers about your plans, where you are hiking to, or if you are planning camping, you can learn more about trail conditions up ahead, blowdowns, or they might let you know the best places to camp. This interaction can benefit you in the case of an emergency; someone would know your whereabouts to direct an emergency crew.

Going to the bathroom: everybody must poop or pee now and again when you're out hiking, especially on that long or overnight hike. One option is to leave your pack on the trail side, not blocking the trail. So you don't pick up any small animals looking for your food stash: the other option is to take your pack with you. The best practice is to go 200 feet away from any water source trail, campsite, or trail to take care of your business. If going off trail is impossible without tramping sensitive vegetation or falling off a cliff, use a little common sense. So that passing hikers are not caught off guard, try to find a private spot behind some trees or rocks.

Hiking, camping, biking, and other forms of outdoor recreation have increased phenomenally in popularity in recent years, and of course, nature calls on all of us. The result is that beautiful places are ruined by waste. Therefore, many scientists and land managers are saying it's time for us to go doo-doo like doggies do: in WAG (Waste Alleviation and Gelling) bags. WAG bags are doggie poop bags for humans; they are a double bag biodegradable system used for disposal in the regular trash. They can be used everywhere and easily make a great addition to your camping gear, hiking pack, or first aid kit. WAG bags are being mandated in many national parks and popular hiking areas. Now the push is to make this the standard practice everywhere.

Depending on whether it's been buried, it can take toilet paper five weeks or more to decompose. Tissues, if thicker than toilet paper, would theoretically take more time. Wet wipes will take around 100 years to decompose, and dog poop bags take around 10-20 years to biodegrade. And please, please, pack out any used toilet paper, poop bags, and sanitary products.

6

Remain on Trail While Hiking

Remain on the trail while hiking. Every American state has sidewalk routes, paved paths, and dirt trails. People Walk, bike, and hike on these trails nearly every day, and they are getting increasingly popular. Paths and trails can be found in national parks, nature preserves, state parks, riverside parks, and just about any other park you can think of. It is important to remember to stay on the trail while enjoying nature, no matter the type of path, mode of transportation, or location.

Staying on the trails is done to protect the people, plant life, and trails themselves. Paths and trails in national and state parks are maintained regularly to ensure they are safe and cleared of obstacles for anyone who wishes to enjoy them. Areas on trails that are prone to washouts can be repaired, excess rocks moved, and trees and shrubs cut back. This is not a guarantee that all trails will be cleared and maintained. After rain or snow storms, the ground can quickly become slippery, muddy, or covered in leaves and twigs. When off trail, a hiker that a natural or unnatural cause had injured would be more difficult to find and assist than if they stayed on a marked, known trail.

Staying on the path is essential even in areas free of trail hazards; wandering off can damage fragile plants and disturb nesting wildlife. Broken branches and snapped limbs are the most obvious signs of damage; not so obvious signs can be young sprouts broken or dug up and prevented from developing into the new plants that keep nature alive. Hiking and riding off the trail could cause damage to the trail, and the compression of topsoil by footprints, tire tracks, or hoof prints can divert water courses during rain and wash out sections of the trail. Rushing diverted water can also cause rocks to be dislodged that become impediments to other hikers on the trail.

Stay on the paths to preserve nature in our parks and preserves and for the safety of others. For your protection and consideration of others and to preserve nature for the future, please keep your boots on the marked paths.

Do not cut switchbacks, no matter how tempting it might be to have a shortcut. When switchbacks are cut over and over, they create side trails causing trail erosion and damage. To prevent damage to the native vegetation along the trail, remain on the trail. Other than trash, leave everything just as you find it. Including any piles of rocks, you might find: these rock cairns have a navigational purpose; building your own or removing ones already there could cause someone else to get lost. Please don't add or remove those strategically placed piles of rocks; instead, leave them be.

Be mindful of trail conditions. If it's early spring, use trails early in the day when they're still frozen. South-facing slopes offer the best conditions when the weather is starting to warm. When natural dirt trails prove too muddy paved trails are an excellent option. Using muddy trails can cause severe, long-lasting, and expensive damage to the trails and surrounding area. Wear suitable footgear so you can walk through the mud, not around it, so you don't damage the vegetation or create side trails. When possible, wait for muddy trails to have time to dry and hike later in the afternoon.

Take time to listen and be aware of your surroundings; turn around and look behind you; you never know what you might see. While hiking, walk quietly, speak softly, and have your cell phone's volume down to off entirely. Carrying a cell phone can be a good tool when hiking. To navigate when needed or in an emergency; however, taking all the calls on your day off is unnecessary. Enjoy the quiet of nature and animals if you see them, and let others do the same. If you use earbuds to listen to music, consider keeping one earbud out so you can hear other trail users who might be coming from behind or trying to communicate with you. Use this same rule when talking on your phone; go ahead and chat, but make sure you are still paying attention to what's happening around you, so you won't miss seeing something that will excite you.

7

Conclusion

Conclusion

Get out and enjoy the many national and state parks we have but remember: Let someone know of your hiking plans. Only take what's necessary for a safe, enjoyable hike to avoid carrying too much weight. Always bring enough water. Choose a trail wisely, do not try a trail that is too difficult to begin with; give yourself time to build up to more difficult levels. Hike with a companion. Remember the "Golden Rule" treat other hikers as you wish to be treated.

If you found this book helpful, I'd be very appreciative if you left a favorable review for the book on Amazon!

www.ingramcontent.com/pod-product-compliance
Lightning Source LLC
Chambersburg PA
CBHW071507150726
48000CB00006B/2730